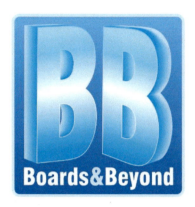

Boards and Beyond: Behavioral Science Slides

Slides from the Boards and Beyond Website

Jason Ryan, MD, MPH

2019 Edition

Table of Contents

Ethics Principles	1	Public Health	16
Informed Consent	5	Quality and Safety	20
Confidentiality	10	The Healthy Patient	27
Decision-Making Capacity	13	Geriatrics	30
		Pediatrics	33

Ethical Principles

Jason Ryan, MD, MPH

Ethics
- Moral principles
- Govern individual or group behavior

Principlism
- Practice of using principles to guide medical ethics
- Most common US framework for ethical reasoning
- Four core principles
  - Autonomy
  - Beneficence
  - Non-maleficence
  - Justice

Autonomy
- Most important US ethical principle
- Absolute right of all competent adult patients to make decisions about their own healthcare
- Patient has "autonomy" over their own body

Autonomy
- Includes right to accept/not accept medical care
- Providers must respect patient decisions
- Providers must honor their preferences

Autonomy
- When patients decline medical care:
  - Okay to ask why they are declining
  - Avoid judging, threatening, or scolding
  - "You may die if you make this choice…"
  - "This choice is a mistake…"
  - "You should not do this…"

Beneficence

- Providers must act in best interests of patients
- Usually superseded by autonomy
  - Patients may choose to act against their interests
  - Example: Patient may decline life-saving medical care

Non-maleficence

- Do no harm
- Always balanced against beneficence
  - Risk versus benefits
  - Some harmful actions (surgery) are beneficial

Justice

- Treat patients fairly and equally
- Also use health resources equitably
- Triage:
  - Form of "distributive justice"
  - Care delivered fairly to all

Gifts from Companies

- Often drug or device companies/manufacturers
- Can influence physician behavior
- Generally acceptable if educational and low value
  - Educational dinner or textbook
  - Value usually should be <$100
- Cash, tickets, vacations, other gifts NOT acceptable

Pixabay/Public Domain

Honoraria

- Fees to physicians paid by industry
  - Goal usually to promote research about a new product
  - Example: Drug company pays MD to speak
- Acceptable but must be disclosed to audience
- Fee must be fair and reasonable
- Fee cannot be in exchange for MD using product

Kolijoriverhouse/Wikipedia

Gifts from Patients

- No definite rules
- In general, small gifts are usually okay
- Large, excessive gifts usually not okay
  - May be viewed as given in exchange for special treatment

Pixabay/Public Domain

Romantic Relationships

- Relationships with current patients never okay
- Per AMA: Sexual contact concurrent with the patient-physician relationship is sexual misconduct

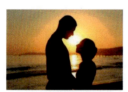

Patient-Physician Relationship

- Physicians may decline to care for a patient
  - Do not have to accept all patients that request care
- Once relationship starts, cannot refuse treatment
  - Example: MD does not want to perform abortion
  - Still must assist the patient
  - Refer to another provider

Medical Errors

- Mistakes/errors should be disclosed to patients

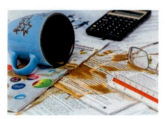

Family and Friends

- Most medical societies recommend against giving non-emergent medical care to family and friends
  - Many ethical conflicts
- Emergencies are an exception

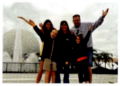

Family of Patients

- May be present during patient encounters
- May answer for patients, disrupt interview
- Don't ask patient if they want family present
  - Patient may be afraid to say no
- Politely ask family for time alone with patient

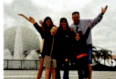

Noncompliant Patients

- Always try to understand WHY
  - Why doesn't patient want to take medications?
  - Why doesn't patient want to go for tests?
- Try to help
  - Provide more information
- Avoid scolding or threats
  - "You will get sick if you don't..."

Emotional Patients

- Acknowledge the patient's feelings
  - "I understand you are upset because…"
- Always try to understand WHY
  - Why is the patient upset?
  - Check for understanding of issues
- Avoid telling patients to calm down
- Don't ignore emotions

Informed Consent

Jason Ryan, MD, MPH

Informed Consent

- All medical interventions require informed consent
- Patient must agree/consent to treatment
- Must inform about benefits, risks, alternatives

Informed Consent

- Benefits
- Risks
  - Must describe all major adverse effects
  - Commonly known risks do not need to be described
  - Example: choking on pill
- Alternative treatments
  - Other therapies
  - What could happen with no treatment

Informed Consent

- Must be in language the patient can understand
  - Must used trained language interpreters
- Must be voluntary (not coerced)
- Patient must have decision-making capacity

Informed Consent

- Patients may withdraw consent at any time

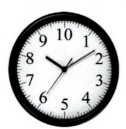

Informed Consent

- Every procedure requires consent
  - Consent for one procedure does not imply consent for another
- Classic example:
  - Mohr vs. Williams
  - Non-life-threatening diagnosis detected in OR
  - Operation for right ear uncovered disease on left
  - Cannot operate left ear without consent
- Emergencies are an exception

Informed Consent
Exceptions

- Lack of decision-making capacity
- Emergencies
- Therapeutic privilege
- Waiver
- Minors

Emergencies

- Consent is implied in an emergency
- Classic example: Unconscious trauma patient

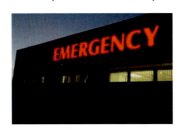

Therapeutic Privilege

- May withhold information when disclosing it would cause dangerous psychological threat
- Often invoked for psychiatric patients at risk of harm
- Information often temporarily withheld until plan put in place with family, other providers

Therapeutic Privilege

- Does not apply to distressing test results
  - Cancer diagnosis would upset patient
  - Family cannot request information be withheld
- Cannot trick patient into treatment
  - Cannot lie to patient to get them to agree to therapy
  - Patient autonomy most important guiding principle

Waiver

- Patient may ask provider not to disclose risks
- Waives the right to informed consent
- Provider not required to state risks over objection
- Try to understand why patient requests waiver

Minors

- Usually defined as person <18 years of age
- Only parent or legal guardian may give consent
- Exceptions
  - Emergency
  - Emancipated minors
  - Special situations

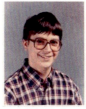

Minors
Emergency Care

- Consent not required (implied)
- Care administered even if parent not present
- Care can be administered against parents' wishes
  - Classic example: Parents are Jehovah's Witnesses
  - Physician may administer blood products to child
  - Do not need court order

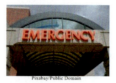

Emancipated Minor

- Minors can attain "legal adulthood" before 18
- Common criteria:
  - Marriage
  - Military service
  - Living separately from parents, managing own affairs
- Emancipated minors may give consent

Minors
Special Situations

- Most US states allow minors to consent for certain interventions without parental consent
  - Contraceptives
  - Prenatal Care
  - Treatment for STDs
  - Treatment for substance abuse

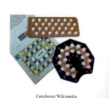

Abortion

- Rules on parental notification vary by state

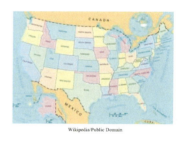

Abortion

- Providers not compelled to perform a procedure
- If patient insists, refer to another provider

Organ Donation

- Brain dead patients are possible organ donors
- In US, organ donation must be discussed only by individuals with specialized training
  - Conflict of interest for caregiver to request organ donation
  - Family may believe physician giving up to obtain organs
- "Organ procurement organizations"
- Often donation coordinator and attending physician

Organ Donation

- In US, individuals assumed NOT to be donors
- Family consent generally required
- Organ donation cards
  - Indicate a preference not final choice
  - Usually not a reason to override family refusal to donate

Moskop J. AMA Journal of Ethics. Organ Donation: When Consent Confronts Refusal. Feb 2003; 5(2)

DNR
Do Not Resuscitate

- Patient request to avoid resuscitative measures
- Meant to decline care in case of cardiac arrest
- No CPR
- No electrical shocks
- Other therapies may still be given
  - Includes ICU care, surgery etc.

DNI
Do Not Intubate

- Patient request to avoid mechanical ventilation
- Often given with DNR: "Patient is DNR/DNI"
- Other therapies may still be given

Advance Care Planning

- Deciding about care prior to incapacitation
- Ideally done as outpatient with primary care MD
- Often done at admission to hospital

Advance Care Planning

- Goal is to identify/document patient wishes
  - DNR/DNI status ("code status")
  - Living will
  - Health Care Proxy
- Very important in patients with chronic illness
  - Cancer
  - Heart Failure
  - COPD

Research

- Research requires consent
- All clinical research studies require informed consent
- Even if drug/therapy is FDA approved
- Even if drug/therapy has no known risks

Research

- Institutional Review Board (IRB)
- Hospital/Institutional committee
- Reviews and approves all research studies
- Ensures protection of human subjects
- Balances risks/benefits
- Ensures adequate informed consent

Research

- Prisoners
  - Informed consent required as for non-prisoners
- Financial disclosures
  - Many companies sponsor research
  - Must inform patients of industry sponsorship

Pregnancy

- Pregnant women may refuse treatment
- Even if baby's health is impacted

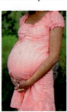
Øyvind Holmstad/Wikipedia

Documentation

- Person performing procedure should obtain and document patient's consent
  - Alternative: someone VERY familiar with procedure
- Often patient asked to sign form
- Act of signing not sufficient for informed consent
  - Patient must be fully informed by provider
  - Patient must have understanding
  - Legal cases have been won despite signed form

Documentation

- Telephone consent is valid
  - Usually requires a "witness"
  - Provider and witness document phone consent

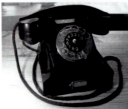
Holger.Ellgaard/Wikipedia

Confidentiality

Jason Ryan, MD, MPH

Confidentiality

- Healthcare information is "privileged and private"
- Providers have duty to respect patient privacy
- Disclosure of patient information should be limited

HIPAA
Health Insurance Portability and Accountability Act of 1996

- Sets national standards for protecting confidentiality
- Identifies protected health information

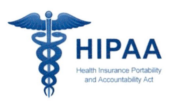

Confidentiality

- Information disclosed only with patient permission
- Includes patient's spouse and children
  - Need patient's permission
- Includes other physicians
  - Must obtain release of information first
- Includes government authorities
  - Unless a court order is issued
- Limited exceptions

Confidentiality

- May tell family a patient's location in ER/hospital
  - "Directory information"
  - Patient location in the facility, general health condition
  - No specific medical information
  - Disclosed if provider deems in patient's best interest

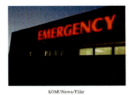

KOMUNews/Flikr

Confidentiality

- May break confidentiality when potential for harm
  - Think: If 3rd party not warned, what will happen?
  - If definite harm ☐ answer is usually to inform

Tarasoff Case

- Tarasoff v. Regents of the University of California (1976)
- Tatiana Tarasoff killed by ex-boyfriend
- Ex-boyfriend treated by psychiatrist at university
- Boyfriend stated intent to kill to psychiatrist
- Authorities notified but not Tarasoff

Public Domain Pictures

Duty to Warn and Protect

- Psychiatric patient intending harm to self/others
  - Suicidal patients (i.e. family notification)
  - Homicidal patients (i.e. police notification)
- Partners of patients with STDs

STDs
Sexually Transmitted Diseases

- Duty to protect/warn partners of patients
  - Partners of HIV+ patients
  - Partners of patients with other STDs
- Only applies to sexual partners
- Does not apply to other individuals
  - Co-workers
  - Students of a teacher
  - Patients of a physician

STDs
Sexually Transmitted Diseases

- Physician may disclose STD status to partners
- May do so without consent in special cases:
  - Reasonable effort to encourage patient to voluntarily disclose
  - Reasonable belief patient will not disclose information
  - Disclosure is necessary to protect health of partner
- Always encourage patient to disclose first
- Some states have partner referral services

www.aids.gov

Reportable Illnesses

- US states mandate certain "reportable diseases"
  - Prevent infectious disease outbreaks
  - Most micro labs have protocols to automatically report
- Tuberculosis
- Syphilis
- Gonorrhea
- Childhood diseases (measles, mumps)
- Many other diseases that vary by state

https://wwwn.cdc.gov/nndss/conditions/notifiable/2017/

Abuse

- Child and elder abuse must be reported
  - Child abuse: Reporting mandatory in all US states
  - Elder abuse: Reporting mandatory in most US states
- Child protective services
- Adult protective services
- Usually history of repeated/suspicious injuries
- First step: child/adult interviewed alone
- Physician protected if reporting proves incorrect

Spousal Abuse

- "Intimate Partner Violence"
- Suggested by multiple, recurrent injuries/accidents
- Primary concern is safety of victim
  - Provider should be supportive
  - May be a difficult topic of discussion
  - Ask if patient feels safe at home
  - Ensure patient has a safe place in emergency
- Some states have reporting requirements

Driving

- Physicians often encounter "impaired drivers"
- Often elderly patients with vision, mobility disorders
- No uniform standard for reporting
- Widely varying rules by US state
- Best answer often to discuss with patient/family

Adam Jones/Flikr

Driving

- Exception: Seizures
- Most states requires a seizure-free interval
  - i.e. 6 months, 1 year
- Often involves consulting with state DMV

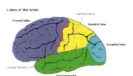

Wikipedia/RobinH

Decision-Making Capacity

Jason Ryan, MD, MPH

Decision-Making Capacity

- Ability to comprehend information about illness and treatment options and make choices in keeping with personal values
- Usually used regarding a specific choice
  - Example: Patient has capacity to consent to surgery
- Required for informed consent
- Key component of ethical principle of autonomy

Competency

- Legal judgment
- Different from decision-making capacity
- Determined by a court/judge
- Clinicians can determine decision-making capacity

Public Domain Pictures

Decision-Making Capacity

- Understanding
  - Patient understands disease and therapy
- Expression of a choice
  - Patient clearly communicates yes or no
- Appreciation of facts
  - Related to understanding
  - Patient understands how disease/therapy affects him/her
- Reasoning
  - Compare options
  - Understand consequences of a choice

Decision-Making Capacity

- Patient is ≥ 18 years old or legally emancipated
- Decision remains stable over time
- Decision not clouded by a mood disorder
- No altered mental status
  - Intoxication
  - Delirium
  - Psychosis

Intellectual Disability

- Patients with Down syndrome, Fragile X
- Does not automatically preclude decision making
- Disabled patient must meet usual requirements
  - Understanding
  - Expression of a choice
  - Appreciation of facts
  - Reasoning

Patients Who Lack Capacity

- Advance directives
- Surrogates

Advance Directives

- Instructions by patient in case of loss of capacity
- Two main types:
  - Living Will
  - Durable Power of Attorney for Health Care

Living Will

- Document of patient preferences for medical care
- Takes effect if patient terminally ill and incapacitated
- Usually addresses life support, critical care
- Often directs withholding of heroic measures

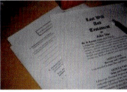
Ken Mayer/Flikr

DPAHC
Durable Power of Attorney for Health Care

- Also called a Health Care Proxy
- Signed legal document
- Authorizes surrogate to make medical decisions
- Surrogate should follow patient's wishes
- Answer question: "What would patient want?"

Absence of Advance Directive

- Some states recognize oral/spoken statements
- Reliable, repeated statements by patient about wishes
- Usually must be witnessed by several people

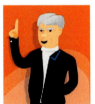
Pixabay/Public Domain

Surrogate Designation

- Used when no advance directives available
- Make decisions when patient loses capacity
- Determine what patient would have wanted
- If no power of attorney:
  - #1: Spouse
  - #2 Adult children
  - #3: Parents
  - #4: Adult siblings
  - #5: Other relatives

Brain Death

- Permanent absence of brain functions
- Brain death = legally dead in the United States
- Life support may be withdrawn
- Even over surrogate/family objections

Public Health

Jason Ryan, MD, MPH

Disease Prevention

- Primary
- Secondary
- Tertiary

Primary Prevention

- Prevents disease from occurring
- Immunizations
- Folate supplementation in pregnancy

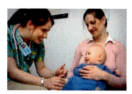

Public Domain

Secondary Prevention

- Prevent disability
- Detect and treat early, ideally when asymptomatic
- Most screening programs
- Mammograms
- Pap smears
- Colonoscopy

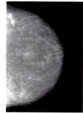

Wikipedia/Public Domain

Tertiary Prevention

- Prevents long-term disease complications
- Maximize remaining function
- Cardiac rehabilitation programs

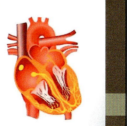

Quaternary Prevention

- Prevents overtreatment or harm from treatment
- Many examples of overuse in US medicine
  - Blood tests
  - Radiology tests
  - Coronary procedures
- Ensure appropriate use

US Healthcare

- Healthcare is expensive ($$$)
- Few patients pay out of pocket
- Major insurance options:
  - Medicare
  - Medicaid
  - Private insurance

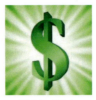

Emergency Care

- Must always be provided regardless of insurance
- After patient stable, insurance can be discussed

Medicare

- Federal program administered by US government
- Paid for by Federal US taxes
- Provides health insurance for:
  - Patients over 65 years of age
  - Disabled
  - Patients on dialysis

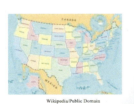

Medicare

- Part A
  - Hospital payments
- Part B
  - Outpatient treatment
  - Clinic visits, diagnostic testing
- Part D
  - Prescription drug coverage

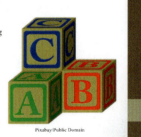

Medicare

- Part C
  - Special option that patients may select
  - Pays private insurer to provide healthcare

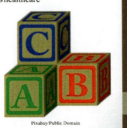

Medicaid

- Jointly funded by state and federal governments
  - Some $$ from Federal government
  - Some $$ from State governments
- Administered by states
- Health insurance for low income patients/families

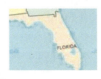 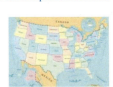

Private Insurance

- Often provided by patient's employer
  - Employer pays fee to insurance company
  - Insurance company pays costs of medical care
- Expensive for employer
- Helps to attract skilled workers
- Several types of plans that vary in features/cost
  - Health Maintenance Organization (HMO)
  - Preferred Provider Organization (PPO)
  - Point of Service plan (POS)

Private Insurance

- Health Maintenance Organization (HMO)
  - Insurance companies hires providers
  - Must use HMO providers - limited choice of physicians
  - Less expensive

Private Insurance

- Preferred Provider Organization (PPO)
  - See any MD you want
  - "In network" MDs have a lower co-pay
  - Most expensive plan
  - Most flexible plan

Private Insurance

- Point of Service plan (POS)
  - Middle option between HMO and PPO
  - Must use specific primary care doctor
  - Can go "out of network" with a higher co-pay

Payment Types

- Fee for service
  - $100 per clinic visit
- Salary
  - $100,000 per year □ doctor must see all patients
- Capitation
  - Set fee paid to physician/hospital per patient/illness
  - Spends LESS than fee □ make money
  - Spends MORE than □ loses money
  - Financial risk transferred to physician/hospital

Affordable Care Act

- Enacted in 2010
- Expands Medicaid coverage
- Establishes exchanges
- Uninsured patients may purchase private healthcare

Hospice

- End of life care
- Focus on quality of life not quantity (prolongation)
- Symptom control
- Services provided at home or in a facility
- Requires expected survival ≤ 6 months

Quality and Safety

Jason Ryan, MD, MPH

Quality and Safety

- Vocabulary
- Hospital Quality Measures
- Prevention and Safety

Care Transition

- Patient transfer
  - Home □ Hospital
  - Hospital □ Home
  - Hospital □ Nursing Home
  - Nursing Home □ Home
- Potential for harm to patients
  - What meds to take?
  - What activates to avoid?
  - When to call doctor?

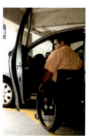

FreeStockPhotos/Public Domain

Medication Reconciliation

- Process of identifying most accurate list of meds
  - Name, dosage, frequency, route
- Done by comparing medical record to external list
- Often done at care transitions
  - Admission to hospital
  - Admission to nursing home

Pixabay/Public Domain

Antimicrobial Stewardship

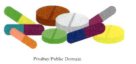

- Hospital program
- Monitors use of antibiotics
- Goals:
  - Prevent emergence of drug-resistant bacteria
  - Promote appropriate use of antibiotics
- Often monitors:
  - Prescribing patterns
  - Microbiology culture results and sensitivities

NIAID/Flikr

SBAR
Situation, Background, Assessment, Recommendation

- Communication tool
- Standardized method of communication
- Often used by nurses when calling MD
- Situation: What is happening
  - Example: Patient has fever
- Background: Who is the patient?
  - Example: Elderly woman with cancer
- Assessment: Other vitals? Labs?
- Recommendation: What is needed?
  - Example: I need to know if you want to start antibiotics.

Quality Measurements

- Readmissions
- Pressure Ulcers
- Surgical-site infections
- Central-line infections
- Ventilator-acquired pneumonia
- Deep vein thrombosis
- Never Events

Hospital Readmission

- Patient X discharged from hospital
- Ten days later, patient X admitted again
- Readmission rate used as a quality indicator
- High readmission rate may be due to:
  - Patient discharged too early
  - Patient not educated prior to discharge
  - Follow-up not scheduled

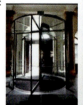

Paul Sableman/Flikr

Hospital Readmission

30-day All-Cause Hospital Readmissions
Most Common Conditions

Heart Failure	Mood Disorders	Chemotherapy	Mood Disorders
Sepsis	Schizophrenia	Mood Disorders	Alcoholism
Pneumonia	Diabetes	Surgical Complications	Diabetes

Healthcare Cost and Utilization Project. Conditions With the Largest Number of Adult Hospital Readmissions by Payer. April 2014

Pressure Ulcers

- Immobile hospitalized patient: ↑ risk skin breakdown
- Can lead to pressure ulcers (usually sacral)
- Causes pain, risk of infection
- Preventative measures
  - Daily skin checks
  - Special mattresses (redistribute pressure)
  - Early identification/care skin breakdown

Pressure Ulcers

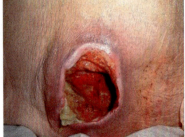

Wikipedia/Public Domain

Surgical Site Infections

- Post-surgical infection
- Often superficial skin infection (cellulitis)
- Can also be deep tissue or organ infection
- Can result from poor sterile technique

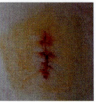

Carsten Niehaus/Wikipedia

Central Line Infections

- Central line insertion can lead to bacteremia
- Can occur due to poor sterile technique
- Gram-positive skin organisms most common
- Staph epidermis and staphylococcus aureus

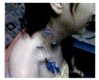
Wikipedia/Public Domain

VAP
Ventilator Acquired Pneumonia

- Pneumonia after patient placed on ventilator
- May be due to hospital factors
  - Failure to elevate head of bed
  - Poor oral care in intubated patients

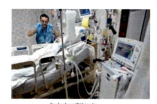
Rcp.basheer/Wikipedia

DVT
Deep Vein Thrombosis

- Immobile, bed-bound patients = ↑ risk thrombus
  - Virchow's triad
  - Stasis, hypercoagulable state, endothelial damage
- ↑ rates of DVT may be due to poor hospital practices
- Methods of prophylaxis:
  - Early ambulation
  - Intermittent pneumatic compression
  - Subcutaneous heparin
  - Low molecular weight heparin (Enoxaparin)

Never Events

- Events that should never happen – no exceptions
- Some examples:
  - Surgery on the wrong site
  - Surgery on the wrong patient
  - Wrong surgical procedure performed
  - Foreign object left inside patient during surgery
  - Administration of incompatible blood

Physician Quality Measurements

- Diabetic patients
  - Foot exams
  - Eye exams
- Systolic heart failure patients
  - ACE inhibitors
- Immunizations

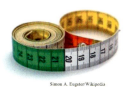
Simon A. Eugster/Wikipedia

Quality Measurements
Process versus Outcome

- Process measurement
  - Rates of immunization
  - Rates of DVT prophylaxis
- Outcome measurement
  - Rates of infection
  - Rates of DVT

Prevention and Safety

- Infection control precautions
- Immunizations
- Root Cause Analysis
- Failure Mode/Effects Analysis
- Time Out
- Checklists
- Triggers and Rapid Response
- Forcing functions/workaround
- Culture of Safety

Infection Control Precautions

- Patients with certain infections need "precautions" taken to prevent spread of disease
- Four basic types of precautions:
  - Standard Precautions
  - Droplet Precautions
  - Contact Precautions
  - Airborne Precautions

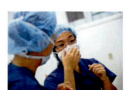

Standard Precautions

- Hand washing
- Gloves when touching blood, body fluids
- Surgical mask/face shield if chance of splash/spray
- Gown if skin or clothing exposed to blood/fluids

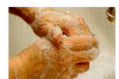

Contact Precautions

- Patients with infections easily spread by contact
- Gloves, gown
- Key pathogens
  - Any infectious diarrhea (norovirus, rotavirus)
  - Especially clostridium difficile
  - MRSA

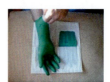

Droplet Precautions

- Patient with infection that spreads by speaking, sneezing, or coughing
- Facemask, gloves and gown
- Key pathogens:
  - Respiratory viruses, especially influenza, RSV
  - Neisseria meningitides
  - Bordetella pertussis

College Student Fever, neck pain

Respiratory Precautions
Airborne/TB precautions

- Patients with infections spread by airborne route
- Fit tested mask or respirator
- Gloves, gown
- Key pathogens
  - Tuberculosis — Fever, cough, Immunocompromise
  - Measles
  - Chickenpox

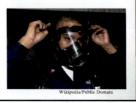

Immunizations

- Many hospitalized patients at risk for influenza and streptococcus pneumonia
- Pneumococcal vaccine
  - Age 65+
  - Age <65 with high risk conditions
  - PPSV23: Contains capsular polysaccharide antigens
  - PCV13: Conjugated to diphtheria toxoid
- Influenza vaccine
  - All persons 6 months and older annually
  - Killed virus vaccine

Root Cause Analysis

- Method to analyze serious adverse events (SAEs)
- Identifies direct cause of error plus contributors
- Example:
  - Wrong drug administered to patient
  - MD error?
  - Nursing error?
  - Labels hard to read: Printing error?
  - Nurses rushed: Hospital error?

Failure Mode & Effects Analysis

- Identifying how a process might fail
  - Root cause analysis done BEFORE adverse event happens
- Identifying effects of potential failure
- Break process down into components
- Look for failure/effect of each component

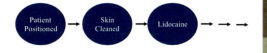

Types of Errors

- Active errors
  - Occur at the end of a process
  - Frontline/bedside operator error
- Latent errors
  - Errors away from bedside that impact care
  - Example: Poor staffing leads to overworked nurses

Swiss Cheese Model

- Flaws at multiple levels align to cause serious errors
- Often more than just a single mistake
  - Institutional factors
  - Supervisor errors
  - Environmental factors
  - Individual error

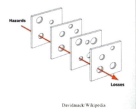

Davidmack/Wikipedia

PDSA
Plan-Do-Study-Act

- PLAN: Plan a change in hospital practice
- DO: Do what you planned
- STUDY: Study the outcome. Did things get better?
- ACT: Act on the study findings
- PDSA "cycles" repeated
- Generates continuous improvement

PDSA
Plan-Do-Study-Act

- Example:
  - Too many surgical site infections
  - Plan to mandate double hand washing
  - Implement plan (Do)
  - Study effects on surgical site infections
  - Action taken based on results

Time Out

- Pause before a medical/surgical procedure
- Patient, physician, nurses, staff all present
- All must agree on patient name, type of procedure

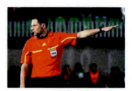

Steindy/Wikipedia

Checklist

- Concept from airline industry
- Series of steps that must be done prior to procedure
- Show to reduce many adverse events
  - Central-line infections
  - Surgical-site infections

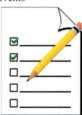

Pixabay/Public Domain

Triggers and Rapid Response

- Patients that "crash" often have signs of impending decline hours before
- Triggers: Patient events that mandate response
  - New chest pain
  - Low oxygen saturation
- Rapid Response Team
  - Provider group
  - Responds to triggers with formal assessment

Forcing Functions

- "Force" an action beneficial for safety
  - Cannot order meds until allergies verified
- Workaround
  - Obtain meds without using ordering system
  - Potential for harm

Human Factors Design

- Design of systems that accounts for human factors
  - How humans work and function
  - How humans interact with system
- Failure to account for human nature ☐ errors

Human Factors Design

- Standardization
  - Same procedures followed throughout hospital
- Simplification
  - Fewer steps → less chance for error
- Forcing functions
  - Cannot only interact with system in one way

Culture of Safety

- Safety as priority for organization
- Teamwork
- Openness and transparency
- Accountability
- Non-punitive responses to adverse events/errors
- Education and training

High Reliability Organization

- Organizations that operate in hazardous conditions
  - High potential for error
- Fewer than average adverse events

The Healthy Patient

Jason Ryan, MD, MPH

Healthy Patients

- Commonly present for "routine evaluation"
- Focus of visit is screening and prevention
- *Criteria for Disease screening*
  - Disease has high burden of suffering
  - Good screening tests
  - Effective early interventions

Cardiovascular Disease

- Several major modifiable risk factors
- Screening and intervention/counseling recommended
  - Diet
  - Obesity
  - Physical inactivity
  - Smoking
  - Hypertension
  - Hyperlipidemia
  - Diabetes

Obesity

Obesity and Body Mass Index (BMI)

$$BMI = \frac{weight\ (kg)}{height^2\ (m^2)}$$

Normal <25 kg/m² | Overweight 25 – 29 kg/m² | Obese ≥ 30 kg/m²

Wikipedia/Public Domain

Obesity

- Behavior modification
  - Mainstay of treatment
  - Make long-term changes in eating behavior and activity
- Drugs (rarely effective)
  - Orlistat (inhibits pancreatic lipase)

Obesity

- **Bariatric surgery**
  - Restricts amount of food stomach can hold
  - Often lead to significant, sustained weight loss
  - Shown to reduce/limit obesity complications (diabetes)
  - BMI > 40 kg/m2
  - BMI 35 – 40 kg/m2 with comorbidities

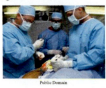

Public Domain

Cardiovascular Disease
Unclear benefit

- Aspirin for primary prevention
- Routine electrocardiogram
- C-reactive protein
- Carotid artery intima-media thickness
- Coronary artery calcification by CT scan
- Homocysteine
- Lipoprotein(a)

Cancer
General Measures

lifestyle as advice.

- Physically activity
- Maintaining a healthy weight
- Healthy diet
- Avoiding smoking
- Limiting alcohol consumption
- Avoiding sexually transmitted infections
- Avoiding excess sun

Obesity

- Excess weight associated with risk for many cancers
- Obesity estimated to cause 20 percent of all cancers
- Absence of excess body fat → ↓ cancer risk*
  - Esophageal adenocarcinoma
  - Colorectal
  - Endometrial
  - Ovarian
  - Pancreatic
  - Postmenopausal breast cancers

*International Agency for Research on Cancer (IARC)

Cancer
Screening

Step 1 won't ask age guidelines

- Breast: mammogram
- Cervical: Pap smear
- Colorectal cancer: colonoscopy or sigmoidoscopy

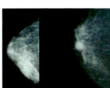
Wikipedia/Public Domain

careful when identifying test for screening v. prevention

Immunization

- Influenza vaccine (all adults)
- Pneumococcus
  - <64 years old if high risk
  - >64 all adults
- Varicella zoster
- Human papilloma virus
- Tetanus, diphtheria, pertussis (boosters)
- Meningococcus (esp. college-age)
- Hepatitis B

STIs
Sexually-Transmitted Infections

- Screening recommended for at risk patients
- Chlamydia and gonorrhea
  - Often asymptomatic
  - Vaginal swab or urine sample
  - Nucleic acid amplification testing (NAAT)
  - Detects organism-specific DNA or RNA
- Hepatitis B
- Hepatitis C (if born between 1945 and 1965) — *remember the blood transfusion issue.*
- HIV
- Syphilis (RPR/VDRL)

Psychosocial Screening

- Depression
- Substance use disorders
  - Alcohol
  - Tobacco
  - Other drugs
- Intimate partner violence

Intimate Partner Violence

- Suggested by multiple, recurrent injuries/accidents
- Primary concern is safety of victim
  - Provider should be supportive
  - May be a difficult topic of discussion
  - Ask if patient feels safe at home
  - Ensure patient has a safe place in emergency
- Some states have reporting requirements

Remember: learned this during the Multiple myeloma week in PBL

Osteoporosis

- All women >65 years old
- Younger women and men with risk factors
- Dual-energy x-ray absorptiometry (DXA)

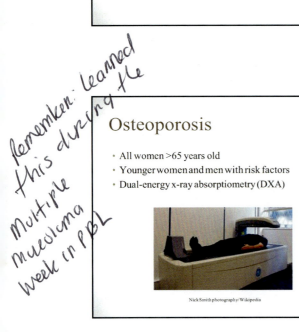

Vascular Disease

- Abdominal aortic aneurysm
  - One-time ultrasound recommended
  - Male smokers ages 65 to 75

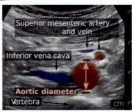

Geriatrics

Jason Ryan, MD, MPH

Geriatric Syndrome
- Group of common health problems among elderly
- Usually multifactorial
- Do not fit in single organ-based categories
- Examples:
  - Cognitive impairment
  - Weakness/fatigue
  - Falls

Public Domain

CGI
Comprehensive Geriatric Assessment
- Functional status
- Fall risk
- Cognition
- Mood
- Polypharmacy
- Social support
- Financial concerns
- Goals of care
- Advanced care preferences

Functional Status
- Basic activities of daily living (BADLs)
  - Basic self care tasks
- Instrumental activities of daily living (IADLs)
  - Tasks required to remain independent
- Advanced activities of daily living (AADLs)
  - Participate in family, social, or work-related roles

BADLs
Basic Activities of Daily Living
- Feeding
- Bathing
- Dressing
- Toileting
- Transferring
- Walking

IADLs
Instrumental Activities of Daily Living
- Shopping for groceries
- Driving or using public transportation
- Using the telephone
- Housework
- Home repair
- Preparing food
- Laundry
- Taking medications
- Managing finances

Pts who can't do this — will need home health aides, or to live in assisted living facilities, nursing homes

Falls

- 50% patients over 80 fall each year
- Many risk factors
  - Prior falls
  - Weakness
  - Balance problems
  - Arthritis
- CNS drugs — Ambien
  - Hypnotics: zolpidem, zaleplon, eszopiclone
  - Benzodiazepines: alprazolam, clonazepam

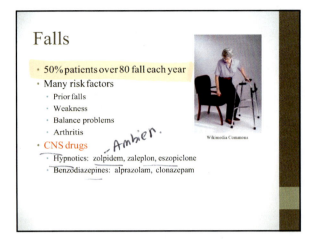

Falls

- Best prevention: exercise
  - Strength training
  - Gait and balance training
  - Tai chi
- Avoid certain medications

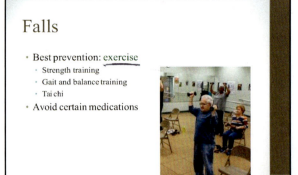

Falls

- Home safety evaluation
  - Stair hand rails
  - Rails in bathrooms
  - Improved lighting
  - Nonslip bath mats
- Walkers/canes
  - May help mobility
  - Little evidence of fall prevention
    - b/c makes pts think they can do more movements and then leads to falls

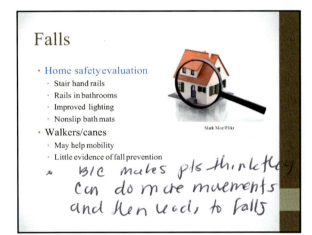

Cognition and Mood

- Cognition
  - Incidence of dementia increases with age
  - Cognition problems often undiagnosed
- Mood
  - Depression very common in elderly
  - Often goes undiagnosed
  - Leads to impaired function, hospitalization

Polypharmacy

- Elderly patients often on multiple medications
- Often have multiple providers (PCP, specialist)
- Review of meds important to prevent med errors

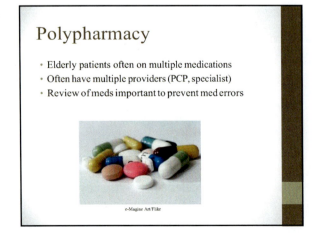

Social and Financial Support

- Strong social support associated with better outcomes
- Elderly often eligible for public financial support
- Caregivers can develop depression or burnout

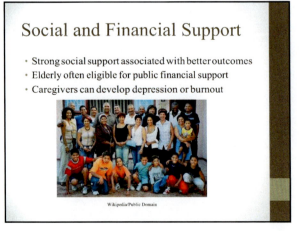

Goals of Care

- Full health and independence often not possible
- Goals of care: What is most important?
  - Living at home
  - Meeting with friends
  - Attending family gatherings
  - Walking without a walker
- What is less important?
- Patients vary in what they value
- Care guided to patient desires

Advanced Care Preferences

- Preferences if health deteriorates
- Especially if patient cannot make decisions

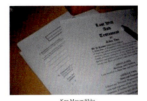

Ken Mayer/Flikr

Remember:
- Healthcare proxies
- Advanced Care Directive at Montefiore
  - End of life care
  - "Do not Resuscitate"

Pediatrics

Jason Ryan, MD, MPH

Labor

- Regular uterine contractions
- Progressive dilation and effacement of cervix
- Descent and expulsion of fetus

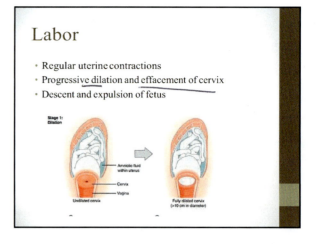

Labor Stages

- Stage I: Onset until cervix dilated 10cm
  - Early Labor Phase: Onset until cervix dilated to 3 cm
  - Active Labor Phase: 3 cm until cervix dilated to 7 cm
  - Transition Phase: 7 cm the cervix fully dilated to 10 cm
- Stage II: Delivery of baby
- Stage III: Delivery of placenta

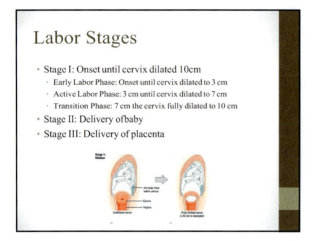

Labor Stages

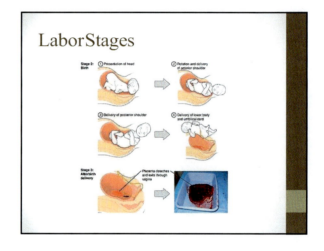

Apgar Scores

- Assigned to children at time of birth
- Assessed at 1 and 5 minutes after birth
- Score of 0, 1, or 2 for the following:
  - Heart rate
  - Respiratory effort
  - Muscle tone
  - Reflex irritability
  - Color
- 90% newborns have scores 7 – 10
- Scores <7 require further evaluation

Apgar Scores

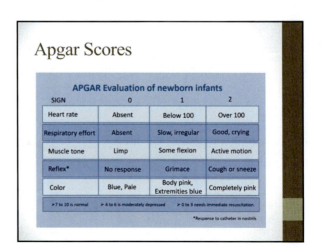

Low Apgar Scores

- Feared outcome: cerebral palsy
  - Most infants with low scores will not develop CP
  - Risk higher with low scores
- 1-minute Apgar score of 0–3:
  - Does not predict outcome
- 5-minute Apgar score of 0–3:
  - Associated with increased risk of neurologic damage

Cerebral Palsy

- Permanent central motor dysfunction
- Affects muscle tone, posture, movement
- Nonprogressive: present at birth and remains
- Caused by damage to fetal or newborn brain
- Can be caused by asphyxia at time of labor
  - Lack of oxygen to the brain

Normal Growth

- Usually occurs in a predictable course
- Influenced by nutrition, health
- Key metrics monitored by pediatricians:
  - Weight
  - Height
  - Head circumference (until 2 years)
- Compared to norms for age group
- Often reported as percentile (10th, 50th, 99th)

Growth Charts
Height, Weight, Head Circumference

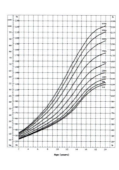

Newborn Weight

- Full term babies lose weight after birth
  - Up to 10 percent of birth weight
  - Occurs in first few days of life
  - Usually regained by 10 to 14 days
- Infants double birth weight by four months
- Triple birth weight by one year
- Children gain ~4.5 lbs per year from 2 to puberty

Linear Growth

- Non-linear with spurts and slowing
- Average length at birth: 20 inches
- Infants grow 10 inches during first year
- Children reach half adult height by 24 to 30 months
- Children grow 2 inches per year ages 2 to puberty
- Normal deceleration of height velocity before puberty
  - Followed by growth spurt

Linear Growth

- Most common causes of short stature after age two:
  - Constitutional growth delay (most common)
  - Familial (genetic) short stature
- Both variants of normal
- Constitutional delay of growth and puberty (CDGP)
  - Late adolescent growth spurt
  - Delayed puberty
  - Adult height often normal

Pathologic Short Stature

- Pulmonary symptoms: cystic fibrosis
- Developmental delay/learning disabilities: Down
- Webbed neck, wide chest: Turner syndrome
- Short limbs compared to torso: achondroplasia

linear those for step!

Head Growth

- Reflects growth of brain
- Small head: microcephaly
- Many, many causes of microcephaly
- Occurs with dysmorphism in many genetic disorders
  - Abnormal facial, limb features
  - Down syndrome (trisomy 21)
  - Angelman syndrome (imprinted gene disorder)
  - Williams syndrome (deletion on chromosome 7)

Down Syndrome

- Birth weight, length, and head circumference low
- Usually remain low until puberty

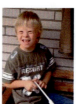
Vanellus Foto/Wikipedia

Developmental Milestones

- Motor, language, and social skills for various ages
- Developmental delay = failure to reach milestones
- Reversible causes:
  - Hearing loss
  - Lead poisoning
- Often occurs with dysmorphic features
  - Facial, limb and other abnormalities
  - Down syndrome
  - Fragile X (long face, large ears, large testes)

MEMORIZE

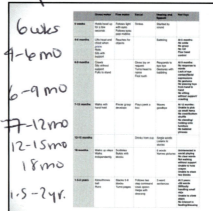

6 wks
4-6 mo
6-9 mo
7-12 mo
12-15 mo
18 mo
1.5-2 yr.

Gross Motor / Fine Motor / Social
Hearing & Speech / Red Flags.

Screening
Select Screening Measures

- Hearing
- Vision
- Iron deficiency
- Lead poisoning
- Oral health
- Tobacco, alcohol, substance use (9 years and older)
- Depression (ages 12 to 21 years)
- Poverty

Iron Deficiency

- Up to 9% toddlers have iron deficiency in US
- Commonly caused by insufficient dietary intake
- Other causes (duodenal absorption):
  - Celiac disease
  - Chron's disease

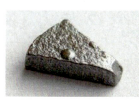
Tomihahndorf

CRAFFT Screening
Substance Use Screen for Children

- Car – Have you ever ridden in a car driven by someone who had been using alcohol or drugs?
- Relax – Do you ever use alcohol or drugs to relax?
- Alone – Do you ever use alcohol or drugs while alone?
- Forget – Do you ever forget things you did while using alcohol or drugs?
- Friends – Do your family or friends ever tell you that you should cut down on your drinking or drug use?
- Trouble – Have you ever gotten into trouble while you were using alcohol or drugs?
- Score ≥2 = high risk adverse outcomes

Car Injuries

- Newborns: rear-facing car seat
- Toddlers/young children: forward-facing car seat
- Older children <12 years: booster seat with seat belt
- Air bags (front seat) dangerous <12 years

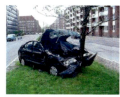
Wikipedia/Public Domain

Poverty

- Screen for lack of basic needs
  - Food, housing, heat
- Providers can link families with community services

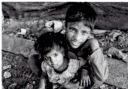
Pixabay/Public Domain

Injuries

- Unintentional injuries: leading cause of death
- Often predictable and preventable
- Car injuries: car seats and seat belts
- Firearms (guns)
  - Gun avoidance (most effective means of prevention)
  - Safe handling and storage of firearms
- Bicycle Injuries
  - Usually head injuries
  - Prevention with bicycle helmets

Anticipatory Guidance

- Given by provider to parents
- Varies by child's age
- Expected growth and development
- Safety reminders

Immunizations

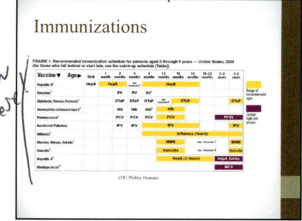

FIGURE 1. Recommended immunization schedule for persons aged 0 through 6 years — United States, 2009

CDC/Public Domain

Puberty

- Transition to sexual maturity
- Two major physiologic events
- Gonadarche:
  - Activation of gonads by pituitary gland
  - Follicle-stimulating hormone (FSH)
  - Luteinizing hormone (LH)
- Adrenarche:
  - Increased androgens from adrenal glands

Puberty

- Thelarche: development of breasts
  - Estradiol action on breast tissue
- Menarche: first menstrual period
- Spermarche: first sperm production
  - Often followed by nocturnal emission
- Pubarche: development of public hair
  - Primarily due to androgens from adrenal gland

Tanner Stages

- Stages I to V
- Assigns stage number to pubertal development
- Separate stages for:
  - Male genitalia
  - Female breasts
  - Pubic hair
- Stage I: prepubertal
- Stage V: adult sexual characteristics
  - Usually occurs by age 15

Tanner Stages

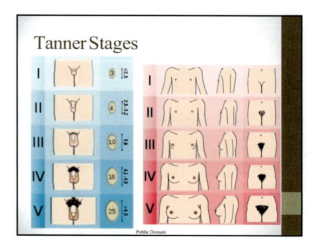

Public Domain

Precocious puberty

- Occurs at early age, usually < 8-9 years old
- Excess androgens (boys) or estrogens (girls)
- Boys: congenital adrenal hyperplasia

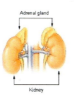

Delayed puberty

- No evidence of puberty by age 12-14 years
- Constitutional delay of growth and puberty
  - Most common cause
- Underproduction of androgens or estrogens
- Hypogonadism:
  - Turner (girls)
  - Klinefelter (boys)
- Kallman syndrome (GnRH deficiency, anosmia)

Made in the USA
Columbia, SC
14 April 2019